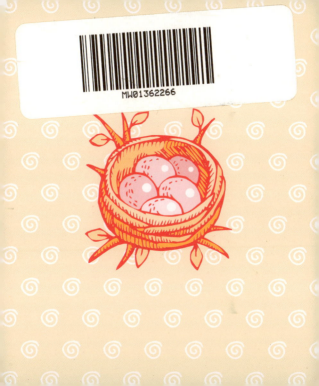

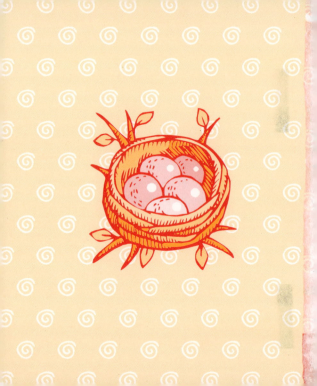

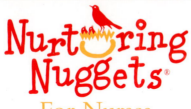

Nurturing Nuggets®
For Nurses

Written by: Susan E. Lanza

Foreword by: Beth Ulrich, EdD, RN, FACHE, FAAN

© 2007 Buttonberry Books
29 Sawmill Road Lebanon, NJ 08833

All rights reserved. No part of this book may be reproduced in any form without the written permission from the publisher.

ISBN 10: 0-9768227-1-7 / ISBN 13: 978-0-9768227-1-4

Printed in China

Book Design by: Peri Poloni-Gabriel,
Knockout Design, www.knockoutbooks.com

Get nurtured at www.NurturingNuggets.com

Foreword

Nursing is a wonderful and rewarding profession full of countless challenges and unending opportunities. As nurses, we are privileged to be present at all the defining moments of people's lives and, through competence and caring, to make each of those moments better.

Nursing isn't easy. In depth knowledge and critical thinking skills are required, and the learning never ends. The hours are often long and the work is hard. But the rewards we get and the joy we feel when we do our jobs well are treasures that few people experience.

In *Nurturing Nuggets for Nurses*, Sue Lanza helps us remember why we became nurses and why we stay in nursing. She also reminds us that we must care for ourselves, as well as for our patients, through honoring our past and each other, celebrating our present, preparing for our future, and balancing our lives.

Nurturing Nuggets for Nurses is a small book, but it carries a major message for nurses. Enjoy!

Beth Ulrich, EdD, RN, FACHE, FAAN

Senior Vice President, Professional Services
Gannett Healthcare Group
Publishers of Nursing Spectrum & NurseWeek
Editor, Nephrology Nursing Journal
BUlrich@GannettHG.com

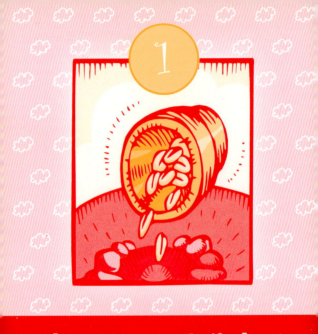

Celebrate Strength In Numbers!

Congratulations RN, you are in good company! There are almost 3 million RN's in the U. S.[1] and nursing has the honor of being the largest health care occupation in the U.S. with approximately 2.4 million jobs held by RN's[2]. Even with those huge numbers, sources estimate that there are currently over 100,000 vacant RN positions within the U.S. alone and by the year 2020, the U.S. shortage of RN's is expected to grow to 800,000[2].

Use your power in numbers to entice newcomers to the profession.

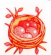

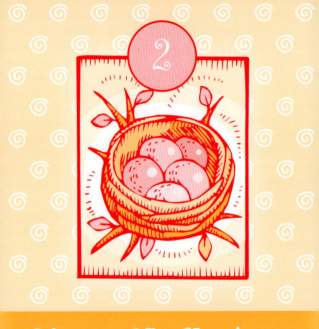

Discover Who You Are

As a nurse, you could be called a "caring scientist" for you combine detailed technical skills with a great compassion to help others. A Registered Nurse treats, manages, and educates patients, along with many other duties. Recent surveys report that the profile of a typical RN is a married Caucasian woman with an average age of 46 who works in a hospital setting[1]. Men still make up a small segment of the workforce. Almost sixty percent of all RN's work full-time.

Statistics define a group but what are your unique characteristics?

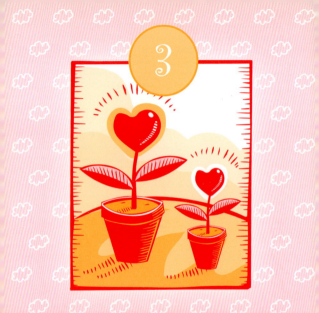

Providing a source of professional identity, the study of nursing history exposes you to critical concepts that help you understand where you fit in as a nurse. From the study of the handling of past epidemics to the examination of how formal nursing training started, these historical investigations enrich your thinking. Florence Nightingale, Linda Richards, Mary Mahoney and Loretta Ford are recognized as some of the esteemed pioneers of modern nursing. So important is the past nursing framework that nursing history is strongly advocated for all levels of training and is a source of continued study by your peers.

Salute your roots!

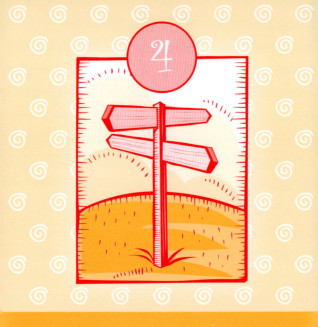

Pioneer Your Path

So what elements of nursing give you joy? Some people know their path before they set foot in school while others "try on" a number of positions until they find their niche. Besides looking into areas of interest, you need to assess your personality and long-range goals:

- Are you outgoing or reserved?
- Do you like detail or prefer broad ideas?
- Do you want to stay in one place or travel?
- Have you set specific objectives for the next 5 years?
- Would you like to manage an organization?
- Do you like to work with a lot of people or be a loner?

- Are you free to work any shift or must you have set hours and times off?

The answers to these questions will help you successfully pick you path. Don't worry if you need to change direction more than once. It is not unusual for nurses to experiment with different areas of the field before getting into a groove.

Knowing yourself will help you with your career path.

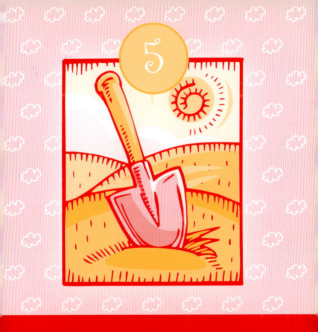

Check Out Fields of Practice

The range of opportunities in nursing is incredible and continues to grow with increasing technology. Although you may have started in one specialty, you have a choice of working within a hospital setting (approximately 60% of all nurses do) or somewhere outside the hospital. In the hospital environment, you can work in broad areas like medical-surgical, labor/delivery, or the operating room. There are a host of sub-specialties, too numerous to list; but they include everything from critical care and hematology to ophthalmology and nephrology. Job specialties are frequently those chosen by:

- population served (e.g., pediatrics or geriatrics)

- type of treatment or work setting (e.g., trauma care)
- disease or condition (e.g., oncology)
- body system or specific organ (e.g., respiratory system)

Outside the hospital walls, the choices are even more varied. You can work in a specific situation like a camp, a school, or in substance abuse recovery, long-term care, or parish nursing. You might also enjoy being an executive, writer, or historical nurse. Or how about military, triage, or forensic nursing?

If you need a change, seek career counseling to find the field for your skill set.

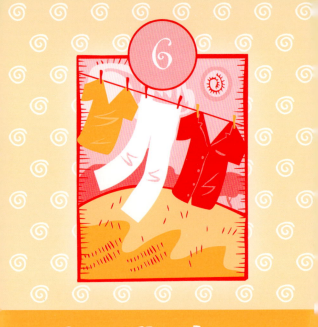

Create Your Look

In nursing today, you find that almost anything goes when it comes to what to wear. Did you think the starched white uniforms were a thing of the past? Not quite. Some nursing schools and employers are returning to traditional whites or choosing a specific color of scrubs as a way to designate the RN's from the crowd. But there are many organizations that give nurses a choice of uniforms and others where no uniform is required. Traditional uniforms started disappearing from fashion in the 1970s and 1980s. One thing every nurse seems to agree on is that wearing a cap is out! The cap, once a symbol of the school you graduated from, has become obsolete.

One of the fallouts in going away from a more traditional white uniform and cap has been that there is no easy way for the public to tell that a nurse is treating them. Some advocates suggest an alternative to the RN uniform by using a patch or pin to let the world know you are a nurse.

How do you express your nursing career with your personal style?

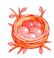

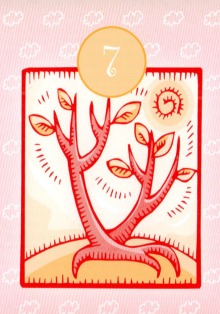

Are You A Nurse In Disguise?

Someone once said "nurses come disguised as many different things." No event brings that statement more in focus than the eleven or more "hidden" nurses who lost their lives on September 11, 2001. You may not have recognized them as nurses because these were multi-talented people who were at the World Trade Center or on the airplanes for many reasons. Among the 11 nurses who perished, there were a number of firefighters from the NYCFD, a Fire Dept. Battalion Chief, two Port Authority Police Officers, an Army Reserve Officer, an Occupational Health Nurse, a Community Health Nurse and a retired nurse. None of them were there in a traditional nursing role, yet their skills were invaluable.

Unseen nurses are everywhere and not so easy to spot since they may not be by the bedside. Valuable skills learned as a nurse are very transferable to other settings such as a running a community organization or working in law enforcement.

Remember that nurses come in many sizes and shapes and do many different things.

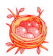

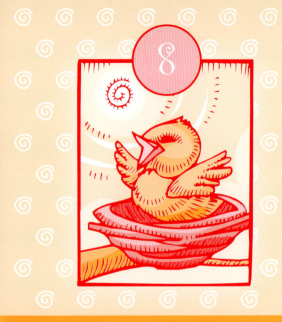

Embrace Opportunities

With an ever-changing marketplace, sooner or later you may find yourself in need of a new nursing position. The good news is that there are many opportunities in nursing. Here are some tips to get you started.

- Determine your long-term career goals.
- Seek career counseling.
- Use library and internet resources.
- Polish your resume and interviewing skills.
- Secure your reference list.
- Know your strengths and weaknesses.
- Network, network, network.

Remember: Leaving one job is an opportunity to begin the job of your dreams!

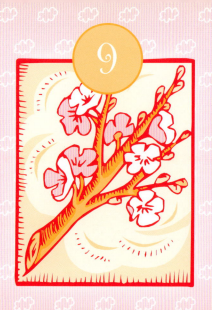

Nurse, Heal Thyself

The physical and mental demands of caring for your patients and your loved ones frequently means less energy left for you to care for yourself. Without a concentrated effort on maintaining your own health, you will find yourself in trouble fast.

Experienced nurses tell us that there are a few simple things that can help you keep yourself healthy. First, stop listening to your inner critic. We take criticism from all sides throughout the day but what about stopping the enemy within? Sometimes you have to figure out the source of the critical voice, forgive yourself and just shut off the negative voices in your head. Other suggestions for healing yourself include staying focused on your goals instead of drifting along with the crowd and feeling resentment later. Simply setting limits and saying "no" to unreasonable requests can make you feel great. Don't forget to make decisions for yourself that reflect your own value system.

Take care of yourself with the same compassion that you take care of your patients.

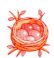

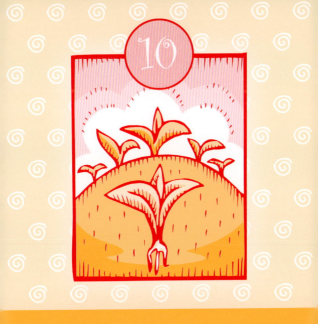

In the process of caring for others, you may forget the significant impact you make on your patients, families and co-workers. A smile or simple thank you from a grateful person can make your day. But what about the times you don't get that feedback? You need to find daily value within yourself. Reflect for a moment on your day. How did your presence make a difference in the lives of your patients and your co-workers? Even on the toughest day, there's always a reason to thank yourself for the special work that you do.

Remember to give yourself mental recognition each day.

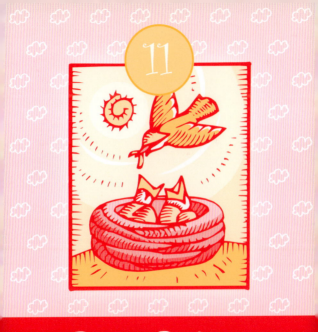

Perfect Patience

One of the top qualities that every nurse is known for is patience. A definition of patience might be the ability to go on with your tasks despite some elements of discomfort or distraction. In fact, the trait of patience joins some of the other core qualities that nurses usually possess including technical competence, patient advocacy, empathy, caring, good communication skills, and professionalism. Patience is tested daily with an environment of fewer co-workers, greater patient loads and sicker patients. Add savvy, demanding consumers to that and this virtue of patience becomes more critical than ever.

Stay as patient as you can be for it is one of your greatest strengths!

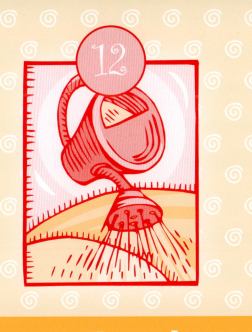

Expand your focus in the career you love by becoming a member of a local and/or national professional organization. Besides getting up to date information, you have your voice heard. Don't see an organization you want to join? Start it yourself, recruiting like-minded nurses to work on your issues or just share social time. Check the internet or your local library to see all the opportunities for meeting your needs.

Being a member of a professional organization will help you thrive.

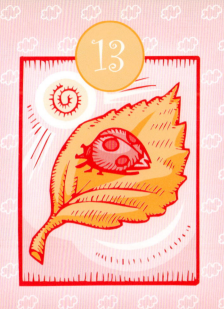

Receive Honors

Kudos to the nursing profession for ranking the highest in yearly surveys of public service professions, year after year. Gallup Poll[3] results show that when various professions are rated on honesty and ethics, nursing professionals are rated number one by the public. Next in line after nurses, are pharmacists, veterinarians, medical doctors and dentists. Such a rating is both an honor and responsibility.

Do your personal ethics and honesty match the poll results?

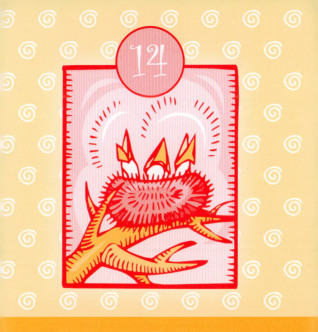

Like any other large profession, nurses who are older, have disabilities or are part of an ethnic minority face their share of unique challenges.

The older nurse, over the age of 50, represents an expanding segment in the workforce and may have difficulty with longer workdays and the sometimes overwhelming physical demands of patient care. Seasoned nurses who face these issues should seek alternate assignments through their employer to help them remain in the profession longer.

Workplace accommodation is also the key for nurses with disabilities. Even with employers making adjustments, the nurse with disabilities may face social and emotional obstacles from misinformed or insensitive colleagues and patients. An advantage that the nurse with disabilities has is special insight and empathy for her patients about being ill and in need of care.

Nurses with an ethnic minority also feel judged on factors that do not relate to their skills. Like their nursing colleagues with disabilities or maturity, minority nurses may feel pressure to prove their value in an often-prejudiced environment.

A new type of workplace barrier has been noted recently as nurses of four distinct age groups have been working side by side with each other. Studies of the multigenerational nurse workforce, which consists of the Veteran Generation (born from 1922-1945), the Baby Boomers (born from 1945-1960), Generation Xers (born from 1960-1980) and the Millennial Generation (born 1980-2000) suggest that knowledge of each group's needs is vital so that teams of different ages can work together harmoniously.[4] The "me" generation Baby Boomers, who are now dominating the workforce, need to find ways to blend with Veterans Generation who are largely rule-abiding and value hard work. The mindset of the Millennial Generation, the next largest group, focuses on their personal contribution and service while the Gen Xers feel very comfortable with technology, but often prefer working in a variety of organizations rather than staying in one place for a long time. Each generation brings its own set of strengths to the workplace. More work is needed is this arena and it is important to note that generalizations about each group are only meant to help other generations understand their needs.

Embrace your fellow nurses for their abundance of skills.

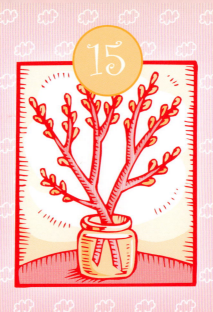

Balance Work & Play

Striking a healthy balance between work life and leisure time may be a challenge for you. Your regular workday is physically and mentally demanding and you often take on extra assignments or stay late. Finding ways to offset this stress is critical. Be sure to include some part of each day that is pure downtime, with no nurse work responsibilities or other big projects.

You owe it to yourself to maintain a balance.

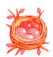

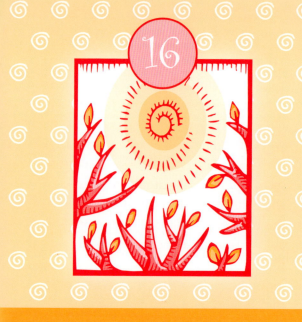

Launch A Second Career

Those who join nursing after another successful career, have qualities that are very attractive to employers. Second career nurses are often determined, having worked while attending another round of schooling. They also share wonderful worker qualities such as emotional maturity, professionalism, and confidence. Recent surveys show that the average age of nursing school graduates continues to climb, pointing to the fact that more students are pursuing nursing following another already successful career[2]. Why this upward trend? Some say that nursing offers a hands-on connection and job satisfaction that few other professions can offer.

Aren't you glad you made the jump into nursing!

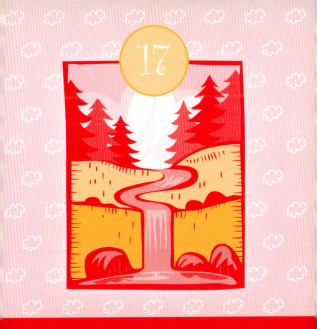

Nursing is one of the exclusive careers that allows for people to come and go, based on life circumstances. If your license has lapsed or you have been out of practice, you need to regain your active status and take a refresher course. Contact your state board of nursing to learn the necessary course requirements and costs. As you reach the bedside for your clinical rotation, expect some normal anxiety. Your course preceptor or supervisor will help you gain confidence to return to the field.

Dust off your skills package and rejoin the work force.

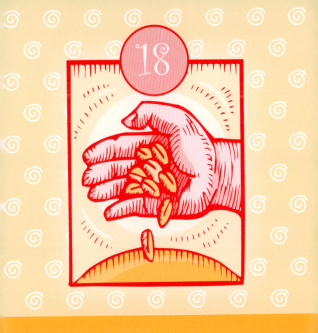

Assess Your Patient Approach

Some nurses define who they are by the simple question, "Do you do direct patient care?" Some nurses interact directly with patients while other nurses might be those in management or educator positions or those in non-direct patient care settings. Don't stoke the differences between the groups but rather, recognize the significant need for both. For example, the oncology nurse works the hands-on side of the case with the patient while the managed care nurse works the indirect care piece; both are important to the patient's health and care.

Accept the contributions of all types of nurses.

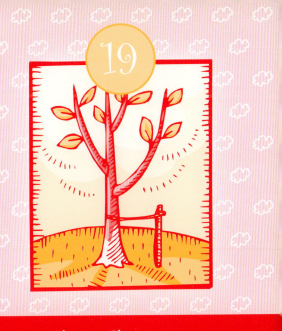

A smart nurse knows when to ask for help, so don't be afraid to let someone know you need assistance. Help may be something as simple as a brief explanation on an unfamiliar topic or as complicated as guidance on handling a conflict. While you were in nursing school or just starting as a professional nurse, you probably were assigned a support person when you were providing patient care. Many nurses maintain relationships with those mentors for years to come. On the job, find a senior colleague who you respect and admire and forge a relationship that will give you the sounding board you may need. Can't find a suitable person? Every healthcare organization has some support staff such as Human Resources so make contact with them for their help with future issues.

Don't be afraid to ask for help!

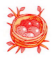

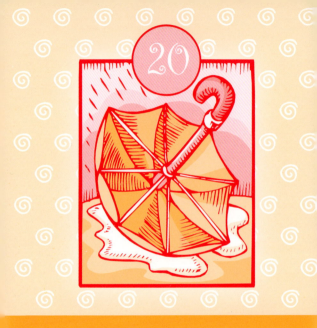

Create Safety

Besides the general occupational hazards of nursing such as standing for long hours, loss of sleep from rotating shifts and on-call status, nurses may face some other unusually dangerous situations. Awareness of potential risks from infections, needle sticks, exposure to chemicals or radiation, exertion injuries, violent patients (or families) and defective equipment should be the focus of any practitioner.

Be smart! Keep yourself and others safe.

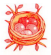

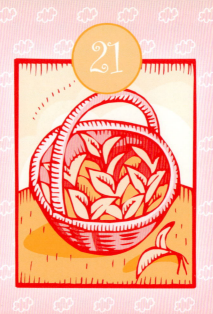
Avoid Burnout

Burnout is caused by overexposure to high levels of stress over a period of time and can be an especially serious problem for people in the caring professions such as nurses.

Every person reaches their burnout point differently, but some of the common symptoms that tell you that you are burning out at your job include: feeling angry or depressed, snapping at co-workers, blaming situations on others, resorting to unhealthy substances (overeating or drug/alcohol use), and having physical signs such as increased blood pressure or headaches. Being in touch with yourself and watching carefully for the first signs of burnout may prevent serious damage to yourself and your patients. Ask a friend or co-worker for an honest review of yourself before things get out of hand.

Maintain your ability to continue caring for others by keeping burnout away.

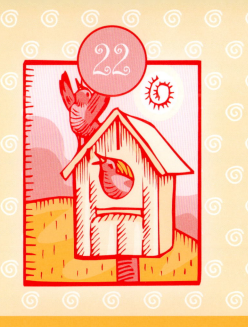

Lead & Mentor

As an RN, you will find that leading and mentoring others can be an interesting and satisfying part of your job. You act as a leader all day by assessing patients, managing staff and families, showing strength and confidence to scared patients, and accomplishing multiple tasks with unending interruptions. Mentoring or guiding others usually happens over time. You may be training new staff and notice that they become comfortable with your approach and seem to come back to you frequently with questions and "what ifs." The next thing you know, you have become a full-fledged mentor, filling the role that was once needed by you. If you want to excel as a leader and mentor, look no further than the writings of nursing pioneer Florence Nightingale[5] whose sage advice holds up in today's nursing environment.

> Instill confidence as you pass your wisdom to others.

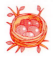

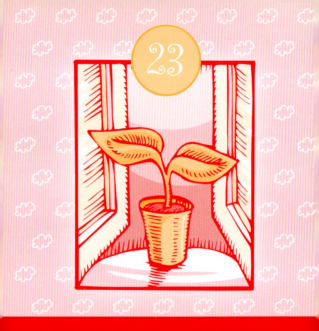

Script Your Future

From your viewpoint, you may say, "What nursing shortage?" as jobs for nurses abound. Nursing employers still struggle to fill key positions, while you have many choices for a bright future. The employment growth rate for RN's is projected to be greater than average for all job types through the year 2014.[2] Some of the occupational expansion will be resulting from technological advances and some from the increasing knowledge base of nurses. Other opportunities will come from the vacancies left by nurses who will be retiring.

Keep the flow of talented nurses coming by encouraging others to join the field.

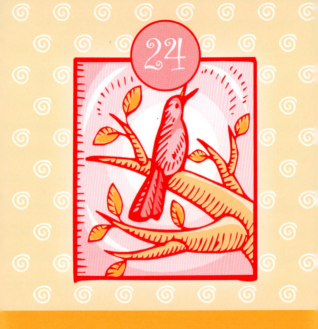

Consider Advanced Practice

When basic nursing education is not enough, aim higher and consider the options of moving into advanced practice or achieving certification. With additional formal education, RN's can become nurse practitioners, clinical nurse specialists, certified nurse midwives, nurse researchers, nurse educators, or nurse anesthetists. All these specialties require a Master's degree or more training.

Certification in various specialties is a nationally sanctioned process that was designed primarily for patient protection. Studies have shown that nurses with certification have a lower rate of errors than those without certification and are more satisfied in general. There are two main types of certification: a certification for minimal standards (you submit your credentials to receive the certification) or a certification for excellence, in which you must demonstrate extraordinary competence in a particular area.

Shoot for the stars and take your career to the next level!

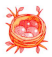

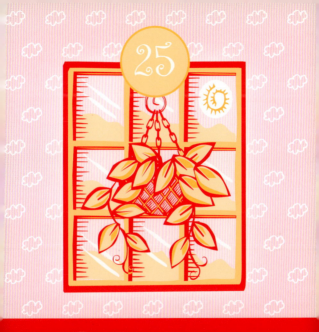

Have you ever said to yourself, "I wish something would change within the nursing profession?" With nursing as the largest health care occupation in the U. S., why not lead the charge and be the change you want to see? The most long lasting transitions in any group usually come from within the group, rather than from an external source. While everyone is sitting around wishing things would change, why don't YOU be the one to get things started? The nursing profession is in need of great leadership and enthusiasm to recruit members to fill the patient needs of the next few decades.

> If you are not the change,
> who will be?

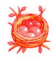

References

[1] National Sample Survey of Registered Nurses (NSSRN), December 2005, U.S. Department of Health & Human Services.

[2] Bureau of Labor Statistics, U.S., Department of Labor, *Occupational Outlook Handbook, 2006-07 Edition*, Registered Nurses, on the internet at http://www.bls.gov/oco/ocos083.htm (August 15, 2006).

[3] The Gallup Poll, December 2006, The Gallup Organization: Princeton, NJ.

[4] Weston, M. J. (2006). Integrating generational perspectives in nursing. *Online Journal of Issues In Nursing*, www.nursingworld.org.

[5] Ulrich, B. T. (1992). *Leadership and management according to Florence Nightingale*. Appleton & Lange: Norwalk, CT.

Resources

General

- Discover Nursing
  www.discovernursing.com
- Minority Nursing
  www.minoritynurse.com
- Nursing Center
  www.nursingcenter.com
- Nursing Schools
  www.allnursingschools.com
- Real Nurse
  www.realnurse.net
- The Center For Nursing Advocacy
  www.nursingadvocacy.org

History

- American Association For The History of Nursing (AAHN) – www.aahn.org

- American Nurses Association Centennial Exhibit: Voices From The Past, Visions of The Future
www.nursingworld.org/centenn/

- Black Nurses In History
www.aetna.com/diversity/aahcalendar/2003/perspective.html

- Canadian Association For The History of Nursing
www.cahn-achn.ca/

- Center For The Study of The History of Nursing
www.nursing.upenn.edu/history/

- Margaret M. Allemang Center For The History of Nursing – www.allemang.on.ca/index.html

- Men In American Nursing History
www.menstuff.org/issues/byissue/nursing.html

- Nurses In The U.S. Navy – Historical Bibliography
www.history.navy.mil/photos/prs-tpic/nurses/nurses.htm

- Nursing History Research Unit At The University of Ottawa
  www.health.uottawa.ca/nursinghistory
- U.S. Army Nurse Corps History
  www.army.mil/cmh-pg/anc/anchhome.html

Organizations

- Academy of Medical-Surgical Nurses
  www.medsurgnurse.org
- American Academy of Ambulatory Care Nursing www.aaacn.org/
- American Academy of Nurse Practitioners
  www.aanp.org
- American Academy of Nurses
  www.aannet.org
- American Assembly For Men In Nursing
  www.aamn.org
- American Association Of Colleges of Nursing
  www.aacn.nche.edu/

- American Association of Critical-Care Nursing
  www.aacn.com
- American Association of Managed Care Nurses
  www.aamcn.org
- American Holistic Nurses Association
  www.ahna.org
- American Nephrology Nurses Association
  www.annanurse.org
- American Nurses Association
  www.nursinginsider.org
- American Nurses Association Hall of Fame
  www.nursinginsider.org/hof/index.htm
- American Nurses Foundation
  www.nursingworld.org/anf
- American Organization of Nurse Executives
  www.aone.org
- Association of periOperative RNs
  www.aorn.org
- American Psychiatric Nurses Association
  www.apna.or

- Association of Rehabilitation Nurses
  www.rehabnurse.org
- Canadian Nurses Association
  www.cna-nurses.ca
- Commission on Graduates of Foreign Nursing Schools – www.cgfns.org
- Emergency Nurses Association
  www.ena.org
- Geriatric Nurses
  www.geronurseonline.org
- International Association of Forensic Nurses
  www.forensicnurse.org
- International Council of Nurses (ICN)
  www.icn.ch
- National Association of Clinical Nurse Specialists
  www.nacns.org/cnsdirectory.shtml
- National Association of Directors of Nursing (NADONA) – www.nadona.org
- National Association of Hispanic Nurses (NAHN) – www.thehispanicnurses.org

- National Association For Practical Nurse Education and Service (NAPNES) www.napnes.org
- National Association of School Nurses www.nasn.org
- National Council State Boards of Nursing www.ncsbn.org
- National Gerontological Nursing Association (NGNA) – www.ngna.org
- National League of Nursing – www.nln.org
- National Student Nurses Association (NSNA) www.nsna.org
- Nurses Christian Fellowship www.ncf-jcn.org
- Nurses Organization For Veteran Affairs www.vanurse.org
- Nurses For A Healthier Tomorrow www.nursesource.org
- Nursing Organizations Alliance www.nursing-alliance.org

- Philippine Nurses Association of America
  www.philippinenursesaa.org

- Sigma Theta Tau International Honor Society of Nursing – www.nursingsociety.org

- Society of Pediatric Nurses
  www.pedsnurses.org

- Society of Trauma Nurses
  www.traumanursesoc.org

Publications

- Advance For Nurses
  www.nursing.advanceweb.com

- American Journal of Nursing
  www.ajnonline.com

- Bio Medical Central
  www.biomedcentral.com

- Evidence Based Nursing
  www.ebn.bmj.com

- Internurse
  www.internurse.com

- Journal of Advanced Nursing
  www.journalofadvancednursing.com
- Journal of Cardiovascular Nursing
  www.jcnjournal.com
- Journal of Holistic Nursing
  www.jhn.sagepub.com
- Journal of Transcultural Nursing
  www.tcn.sagepub.com
- Nurseweek
  www.nurse.com
- Nursing Spectrum
  www.nurse.com
- RN Web
  www.rnweb.com
- RN Week Magazine
  www.rnweek.com

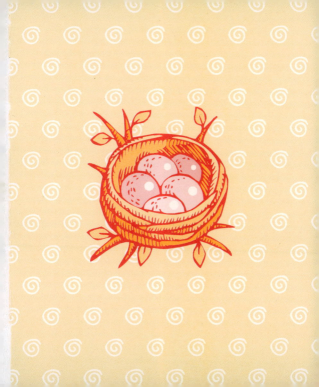

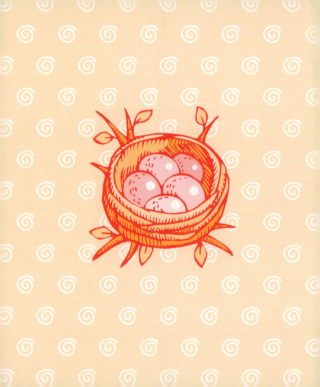